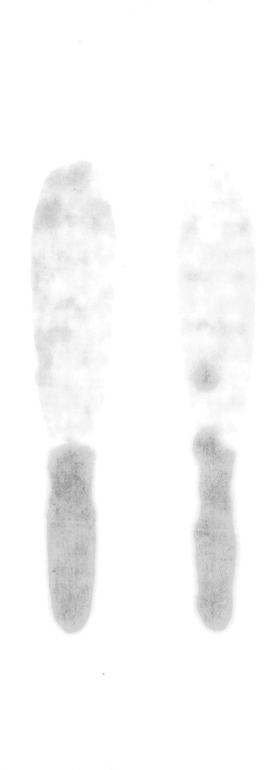

ADVICE TO PARENTS

OF A CLEFT PALATE CHILD

ADVICE TO PARENTS

OF A CLEFT PALATE CHILD

Second Edition

By

DONNA KONKEL WICKA, M.A.

Troy Public Schools
Troy, Michigan

and

MERVYN L. FALK, Ph.D.

Department of Speech
Communication Disorders and Sciences
Wayne State University
Detroit, Michigan

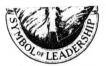

CHARLES C THOMAS • PUBLISHER
Springfield • Illinois • U.S.A.

Published and Distributed Throughout the World by

CHARLES C THOMAS • PUBLISHER
2600 South First Street
Springfield, Illinois, 62717 U.S.A.

© *1982 by* CHARLES C THOMAS • PUBLISHER

ISBN 0-398-04704-9

Library of Congress Catalog Card Number: 82-3260

*With THOMAS BOOKS careful attention is given to all details of
manufacturing and design. It is the Publisher's desire to present books that are
satisfactory as to their physical qualities and artistic possibilities and
appropriate for their particular use. THOMAS BOOKS will be true to those
laws of quality that assure a good name and good will.*

Printed in the United States of America
I-AM5-1

Library of Congress Cataloging in Publication Data

Wicka, Donna Konkel.
    Advice to parents of a cleft palate child.

    Bibliography: p.
    1. Cleft palate--Surgery.   2. Cleft palate--Psycho-
logical aspects.   I. Falk, Mervyn L.   II. Title.   [DNLM:
1. Cleft palate--Popular works.   2. Child care--Popu-
lar works.   3. Parent-child relations--Popular works.
WV 440 W636a]
RD525.W5 1982   618.92'097522   82-3260
ISBN 0-398-04704-9   AACR2

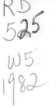

PREFACE TO THE SECOND EDITION

IN THE TEN YEARS THAT HAVE ELAPSED SINCE OUR ORIGINAL PUBLICATION, NOTEWORTHY ADVANCEMENTS HAVE OC-curred in managing the various disorders that accompany cleft lip and palate.

In our effort to present to parents of the newborn with oral cleft a comprehensive overview of the meaning of this problem to them as well as to their child, it becomes important to update this information and to improve, as well, our original presentation.

We have, therefore, significantly altered the chapter on the speech disorder that often accompanies oral cleft and have made an attempt to provide added insight regarding parental involvement in normal language development.

The reader will find that materials have also been refined in the chapters that address the medical and dental management of this disorder.

The nature of the difficulties created by oral clefting do not seem to have changed; we would hope, however, that insight, skill, and dedication with regard to this anomaly have significantly improved treatment since our last writing.

D.K.W.
M.L.F.

PREFACE TO THE FIRST EDITION

MOST PROFESSIONALS AGREE THAT THE PARENTS OF CHILDREN WITH CLEFTS NEED A GREAT DEAL OF COUNSELING and advice. Koepp-Baker states, "The parents must be helped to understand the child's problems, the details and nature of his medical, dental, surgical, and speech care" (23, p. 606). Tiesza and Gumpertz's opinion is the same as Koepp-Baker's: "The parents need understanding, concrete hope, practical advice, and considerable anticipatory guidance concerning feeding, speech and community facilities"

(52, p. 99).

The purpose then of this book is to serve as a source of information for the parents of a child with a cleft palate and/or lip. The work of many professionals in the area of cleft palate has been reviewed and summarized in order to present a comprehensive study of the disorder. It is our hope that this book will give parents a better understanding of what cleft palate means for the future of their child.

We wish to express our appreciation to Karen A. Green for her help in the final preparation of this manuscript.

D.K.W.
M.L.F.

CONTENTS

ADVICE TO PARENTS

OF A CLEFT PALATE CHILD

Chapter 1

THE INCIDENCE AND ETIOLOGY

OF CLEFT PALATE

P ROBABLY ONE OF THE FIRST QUESTIONS THAT OCCURS WHEN PARENTS ARE IN- FORMED THAT THEIR CHILD HAS A CLEFT palate is "What causes it?" Therefore, the first area to be con- sidered in the discussion of cleft lip and palate will be its in- cidence and etiology.

Statistics on the occurrence of clefts vary in the literature from 1 in 600 to 1 in 1000 births (12). It can be said that approximately one baby in every 750 will be born with a cleft lip and/or palate; an apparent increase over past years. This rise in the number of children with clefts can be attributed to two factors. First, better methods have been established for keeping track of such statistics. It has only been recently that laws have been established in some states requiring physicians to report such congenital anomalies. Second, the mortality rate in cleft palate children has decreased due to a greater percentage of conceptions being successfully brought to term and to a decrease in the nutritional and surgical problems encountered.

Research indicates that there are more Caucasian than Negro children born with clefts. Approximately 4 out of every 100 cleft palate births are nonwhite, while the ratio is 10 to 100 for nonwhite births in the general population. More males are born with clefts than females with a ratio of about three boys to every two girls. It is further reported that clefts of the palate alone occur slightly more frequently among females, while clefts of the lip alone occur more frequently among males. Data also indicate that some type of oral cleft occurs twice as often in multiple births as in single births. Incidence is reported of 2.2 percent among multiple births and 1.0 percent in the general population.

No one has established the cause or causes of oral clefts, but, at present, several theories exist that can be grouped into three broad categories: (a) intrauterine difficulty during the first three months of pregnancy until the palate of the embryo has fused, (b) mechanical obstructions, and (c) heredity.

The following are some of the maternal factors that produce an unfavorable environment and might prevent proper fusion of segments in the embryo:

1. Malnutrition.
2. Vitamin A in excess or deficiency — cleft lips and palates have been produced in experimentation with

rats by depriving them of vitamin A.

3. Cortisone therapy.
4. Insulin injection.
5. Rubella and possibly other virus infections such as mumps.
6. Toxemia of pregnancy.
7. Pernicious vomiting during pregnancy.
8. Anoxia (lack of oxygen in the blood).
9. Radiation.

Mechanical obstructions include uterine tumors, cord interference, pressure of the lower jaw, and interference of the hands and feet. It is also felt by some that a cleft could be caused by a failure of the tongue to descend from the nasal cavity.

Hereditary factors appear to account for approximately 30 percent of all cases of oral cleft. It is believed that a particular recessive gene is responsible for transmitting the problem. It is of interest, however, that all babies who inherit the gene do not suffer from the deformity. It is likely, therefore, that additional influences exert their effects before deformity becomes manifest. In general, when either parent or a sibling suffers from a facial cleft, the unborn child has a 5 percent chance of a similar handicap; when both a parent and a sibling are affected, the risk rises to 15 percent (38).

One author (14) states that there is no genetic relationship between an isolated cleft palate and a cleft lip with or without cleft palate. Therefore, a parent with a simple cleft palate or normal parents with a child with a cleft palate can be assured that there is no genetic basis for a cleft lip occurring in the family.

When a man or woman with a cleft lip marries a normal partner, the chance of their child having a cleft is 2 percent. With cleft palate the situation is a little different. In that case, a parent with a cleft is very unlikely to have a deformed child, unless he or she has several relatives afflicted, in which case the risk increases. When the normal parents of a child with a cleft seek advice concerning further children, the risk may be stated as 2 percent for cleft lip and 4 percent for cleft palate.

First children are no more or less prone to the condition than any other numbers in the family series, nor does the age of the parents in any way increase the danger. However, if one of the parents has a cleft lip or palate, the appearance of the lesion in their child carries a 15 percent risk of its recurrence in further children (12).

In conclusion, it can be stated that one in about every 750 children has a cleft lip and/or palate, with more of these being boys than girls. A cleft can be caused by unfavorable maternal environment, by a mechanical obstruction, or through heredity. Heredity is presumed to be a causal factor in only approximately 20 to 30 percent of all cleft cases.

Chapter 2

THE SPEECH CHARACTERISTICS OF

A CHILD WITH CLEFT PALATE

T HE SPEECH AND LANGUAGE PATTERNS OF THOSE BORN WITH CLEFT LIP AND/OR PALATE, AS IN THE GENERAL POPULA-tion, can range from normal to severely impaired. Though speech may be one of the cleft patient's most serious problems, it can, in most cases, be corrected through any combination of appropriate training, surgery, and dental management.

Investigations have found that individuals with the singular problem of cleft lip have essentially normal articulation skills, while individuals with lip and palate clefts demonstrate a higher level of articulation skill than do individuals with only palatal clefts. This suggests that the ability to close the palate and maintain oral pressure is an important factor in the articulatory proficiency of children.

Articulation errors, that is the inability to produce sounds correctly, and nasality are the two most frequent and significant communicative problems of speakers with cleft palates. Of the two, articulation errors are felt to be the more detrimental to effective communication (31).

As stated before, the inability to close off the nasal cavity from the oral cavity is the principal factor in accounting for articulation errors and nasality.

In order to understand how a palatal cleft can cause problems in speaking, it is important to know how normal speech is produced.

Air is allowed to escape from the lungs, pass through the vocal cords, and enter the oral cavity. The position of the tongue, lips, lower jaw, and soft palate working together in a highly coordinated fashion results in the sounds of speech being produced. If the vocal cords are set into vibration while the airstream is passing between, then voice is superimposed upon the speech sounds that result from the relationships of the oral structures. While the soft palate is raised during speech production, air is prevented from escaping through the nose.

Of forty-five speech sounds in the English language, only three are normally produced with the soft palate lowered. The sounds m-n-ng result from nasal airflow in normal speech production; all remaining sounds are produced with the soft palate in contact with the pharynx at a level above the hard and soft palates.

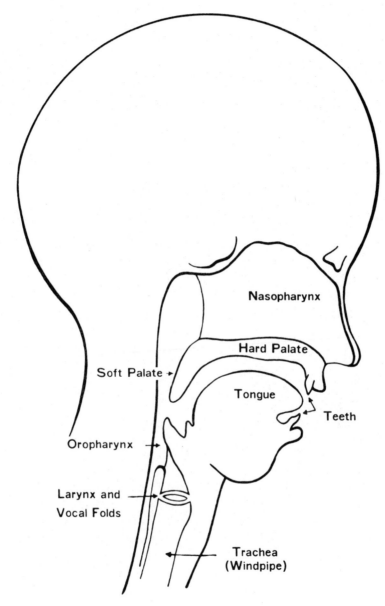

Figure 1. Illustration of the speech mechanism.

This brief description of normal speech production can be contrasted with what occurs in the presence of a deficient palate. If either the hard or soft palate is cleft or if the soft palate is either short or immobile, air is permitted to enter into the nasal cavity for sound production other than those sounds normally produced through the nose.

With improvements made in surgical repair during the past ten years, many children are now seen who have very adequate anatomy for normal speech production, yet still speak with nasality due to the articulation patterns acquired prior to surgery. These children respond to articulation therapy that is designed to establish normal production of the defective speech sounds, which , in turn, eliminates the nasality.

For some time, speech of the cleft palate child develops along lines similar to a normal child. Early vocalizations of the child with a cleft are about the same as those of other children in amount and intent. Children with clefts, however, are slower to develop clear sounds. They use fewer consonants, lack variety in both vowels and consonants, and rely heavily on sounds that can be produced in the back of the mouth (40).

Some patients with cleft palate have little or no trouble in producing intelligible speech, while others have many and severe types of misarticulation, including omissions, substitutions, additions, and distortions of speech sounds, that interfere with their ability to produce acceptable, understandable speech (44).

Children who have cleft lip without cleft palate usually have very few articulation problems. When they do, however, their difficulties are usually with sounds formed by one or both lips such as p, b, m, f, and v. Distortions of these sounds may be due to immobility of the lips either from habit, extreme surgical repair, or missing teeth (44).

One study of the articulation patterns of children with cleft palates between the ages of three and seven years found that cleft palate children are less proficient in articulation skills than are noncleft palate children (1). The five-year-old cleft palate children in this study were less proficient in articulation than were the three-year-old normals. Consonant blends such as sk and sl, fricatives such as f, s, and sh, and plosives such as p and b were relatively more difficult for the cleft palate subjects. Also, the young cleft palate children were more proficient on the voiced consonant sounds than on their voiceless cognates. They were least proficient on sounds in the medial positions in words.

The same study also concluded that cleft palate children make substitution errors more than twice as frequently, distort sounds more than twice as frequently, and omit sounds almost four times as frequently as noncleft children.

Another study (34) investigated the articulation skills of twenty-five children with cleft lips and palates from the ages of three to eight years.

It was found that these children had little difficulty with vowels or diphthongs, producing them correctly 96 percent of the time. The consonants they misarticulated more than 60 percent of the time were z, th, s, ch, zh, j, sh, and t. The five consonants giving them the least difficulty were m, n, h, y, and ng. When compared with noncleft children, this group seemed to be generally behind in articulation skills.

Studies (6, 20) have also examined the articulation skills of adults with cleft palates. Results have indicated that about 70 percent of consonants are produced correctly with s, z causing the most difficulty. Nasal emission appeared to be a significant factor in these misarticulations.

The differences in number of misarticulations between children and adults with repaired cleft palates show that, with proper management, the speech of a cleft palate child can be greatly improved.

For speakers with cleft palates, difficulty with articulation of sounds can be caused by several factors:

1. inadequate intraoral breath pressure as a result of velopharyngeal incompetence
2. deformities of the lips and deviations of the teeth and and dental arches
3. functional misuse of the tongue
4. hearing loss

Besides the four basic causes for articulation difficulties, one author states: "A most important factor influencing articulation patterns in children with cleft lip and palate is the manner in which they receive early language and speech stimulation from family, friends, and teachers. Many articulation problems grow out of the child's compensatory actions when well-meaning but oftentimes misguided parents and teachers urge him to make his speech clear. The resulting overenergized attempts to produce clear speech sounds become incorporated into his everyday speaking habits" (44).

Questions often arise concerning the language ability of children with cleft palate. Language is defined as a means of expression and communication. Most authorities agree that these children are usually somewhat slower in developing language skills. It is felt that the cause of this slowness is not due to any intelligence factor, but because they may be shy and withdrawn due to their articulatory difficulties.

There is also evidence that suggests that, as a group, these children are immature in length of responses and vocabulary usage. This is attributed to the fact that they probably do not find speech as pleasant, satisfying, or rewarding as do children without clefts and, therefore, talk less. They are not, however, different from noncleft speakers in the structural complexity of their speech.

It is generally agreed that children with cleft lip and palate are as intelligent as their peers and have substantially equal language development, but may not be as expressive as are their noncleft counterparts. Their tendency toward shorter utterances, however, may be attributed to their self-concept rather than to a real lack of ability to express themselves.

It is important to mention here that most children with a cleft palate who are delayed in language development eventually do catch up to other children of the same age group if adults require them to make an attempt to verbalize rather than depending on gestures to communicate.

In summary, then, speech has been found to be one of the major problems encountered by those having a cleft, with misarticulations and nasality being the areas of greatest difficulty. The sounds found to be most often misarticulated by those with clefts are z, th, s, ch, zh, j, sh, and t.

Chapter 3

FEEDING MANAGEMENT

AND ITS IMPLICATIONS

FOR SPEECH DEVELOPMENT

A LTHOUGH THE PEDIATRICIAN IS DIRECT-
LY RESPONSIBLE FOR THE FEEDING
MANAGEMENT OF THE CHILD WITH A
cleft, the speech clinician is also concerned because of the
implications feeding techniques hold for later speech development.

Speech is often called an overlaid function because there
are no speech organs as such. The tongue, jaws, lips, and
palate are primarily organs for the chewing and swallowing of

food. The vocal folds function primarily as a valve to protect the windpipe and lungs from material other than air taken into the mouth. These functions are reflexive in nature. Nevertheless, these same structures are also used in speech production. A child must learn to adapt the basic functions of these structures and coordinate the movements of the various muscle groups in order to produce speech.

When an infant who has an intact lip and palate sucks, the area between the nasal and oral cavities remains open and the child continues to breath through the nose, alternating with or simultaneous to the sucking. The soft palate is lowered somewhat and rests on the back of the tongue. The lips enclose the nipple and seal the entrance to the mouth, the nipple being held and compressed between the tongue tip and alveolus (gums). By lowering the floor of the mouth, a negative pressure is created and fluids are drawn into the mouth.

"When the alveolus and lip are cleft, the tongue tip will fail to experience normal contacts and resistance, as when attempting to compress the nipple. Compensatory adjustments are developed, and sensori-motor experience must necessarily differ from that of the child with a normal palate. These compensations may later affect the use and development of certain articulatory movements for consonant sounds post-operatively" (24, p. 47).

The ability to make sounds and words in speech (articulation) is "an acquired motor skill developed gradually in childhood and dependent on the normal functioning of the motor system for the muscle movements and coordinations required. . ." (24, p. 51).

In a child with a cleft palate, these movements and coordinations differ from the normal child. Compensatory movement patterns are developed to maintain the ability to suck. For example, to achieve negative oral pressure for sucking, the child may raise the back part of the tongue in an attempt to close the cleft. The infant's use of his tongue and lips during vocal play may be influenced by these compensatory adjustments, and later even articulation of speech sounds may be affected (24).

Babies with cleft lip and palate generally start to suck when a nipple is placed in their mouth just as any newborn baby does. This occurs because the sucking and swallowing reflexes are present, even though the muscles are not able to operate as efficiently as they should. It is important that these muscle movements be developed as early as possible, not only to assure proper eating, but also for the baby's later speech development.

Ordinarily, the larger the cleft, the larger the nipple should be in size so that the baby can grasp it successfully. It should be inserted further back in his mouth than would usually be done in infant feeding. The holes in the nipple will need to be larger. If persistent attempts to feed with a bottle and nipple fail, then a special type of feeder may have to be used.

One type of nipple frequently used is called a lamb's nipple. This is larger than the ordinary nipple and has a bigger hole. Because of its tapered shape and size of hole, the infant is able to feed with a minimum of sucking (3).

More recently, it has been found that providing the infant with a prosthesis has increased the proportion of patients who can feed on the breast or by bottle. Instead of having to be fed frequently and laboriously with a teaspoon or special feeding bottle, many patients can now suck and swallow almost normally. Not only has this greatly simplified the feeding problems of patients, but it has probably allowed many of them to develop tongue and palatal movements in the course of feeding like those of normal children (9). As stated before, it is felt that these sucking movements, even though very basic, are of greatest importance in the development of speech.

In conclusion, it can be stated that proper feeding is important for children with clefts, not only for nutritional purposes but also because the structures used in chewing, sucking, and swallowing are also used in speech. Often, larger holes are needed in the nipple or a larger nipple is necessary. Special feeders, such as a lamb's nipple, may be needed in some cases.

Chapter 4

PLASTIC AND RECONSTRUCTIVE

SURGERY

IN MOST CASES, LIP REPAIR IS THE FIRST STEP TOWARD HABILITATION OF THE CHILD WITH A CLEFT LIP AND PALATE. There is some controversy as to when the ideal time for such surgery exists, although most surgeons agree that it should be within the first six months of life (43). The surgeons at St. Luke's Hospital Cleft Palate Clinic suggest for the following reasons that repair take place during the first week of life:

1. A very young infant has immunity from the mother and a high resistance to infection, therefore, can tolerate surgery well and require a minimum of anesthetic.

2. The cleft lip can cause difficulties in sucking that can be remedied by early surgical intervention, causing growth and weight gain to progress at a normal rate.

3. Early repair of the nonunited lip muscles will provide a biological orthodontic band that exerts a powerful molding action upon the cleft maxillary segments. This molding action will help to narrow the palatal cleft somewhat (7).

Proponents of later surgery feel that the size of the lip in a newborn makes accurate repair difficult. They feel that it is better for the baby's health if he is permitted to gain weight before he undergoes surgery (7).

There are many different techniques used in lip repair. The degree of involvement of the lip, nose, and alveolus (primary palate) varies greatly and largely determines the method of repair employed in each case (7). Type of repair depends upon what appears to be best suited to the individual patient and upon the favorite technique of the surgeon.

The aims of initial lip surgery are to bring together the separated parts of the lip in such a fashion as to provide the child with as normal an appearance to the lip and nose as is possible and also to aid in the development of normal lip function. In bringing the lip together, the surgeon strives for a symmetrical lip with a natural appearing midportion (cupid's bow), a fullness to the red portion of the lip (vermilion), with preservation of the white line, a natural appearing vertical depression between the lip and nose (philtrum), and a symmetrical nose with restoration of the nostril floor and nasal tip.

In some cases, when the cleft is slight, the goals of the surgeon can be achieved through initial surgery (7). In other cases, however, there may be need for secondary surgery of the lip and nose.

The purpose of secondary plastic operations is to improve the relationship of the facial parts in order to make them more normal in appearance. Oftentimes it is necessary to improve the location of the cupid's bow, which is sometimes found displaced toward the side of the cleft, or to improve the relation between maxilla and mandible. Other defects that may later call for correction are an irregular, overly full, or notched inferior margin of the upper lip; a tight lip lacking a rounded profile and natural pout; absence of the philtrum; or a widened scar (37).

Of vital importance to the child with a cleft is the repair of the palate. Stark states that "A cleft of the secondary palate is a considerable handicap because an incompetent velopharyngeal valve results in defective speech and deglutition and, in some cases, defective hearing. A cleft that traverses the alveolus as well (cleft of the primary and secondary palates) affects dentition, both functionally and cosmetically, and articulation may be faulty. Because of these inherent problems, initial cleft palate surgery has many goals" (36, p. 153).

The main purpose of palate surgery is to construct an intact and mobile palate that can operate efficiently in closing off the nasal cavity, thus permitting the airstream for speech to be directed through the oral cavity and food to be directed into the esophagus. Secondary goals are the preservation of normal development of the bony growth of the central face and functional dentition (36).

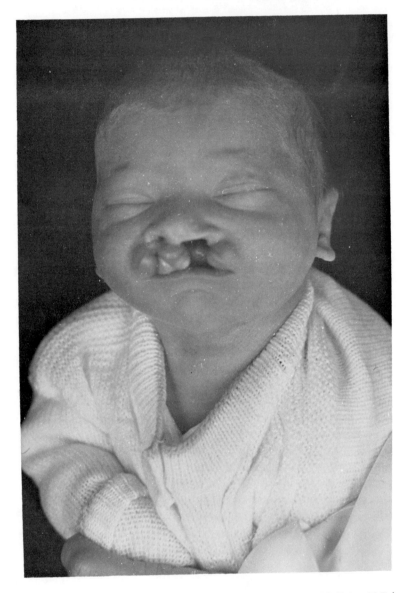

Figure 2. Unrepaired bilateral cleft lip. (Courtesy of W. E. McEvitt, M.D.)

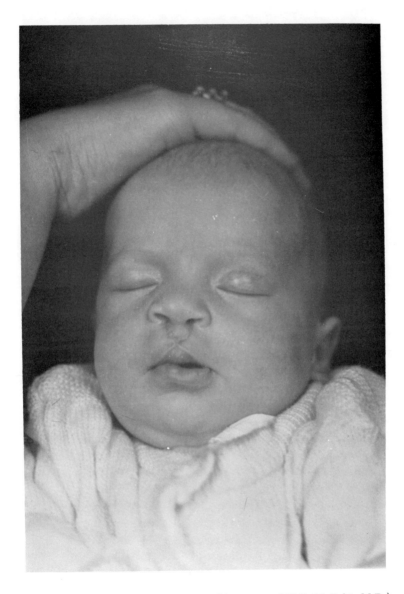

Figure 3. Repaired bilateral cleft lip. (Courtesy of W.E. McEvitt, M.D.)

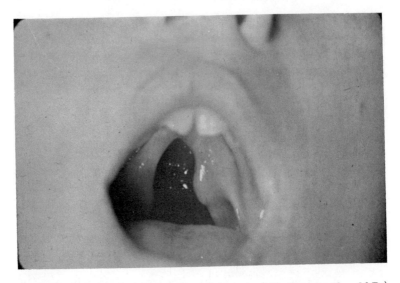

Figure 4. Unrepaired cleft palate. (Courtesy of D. Kapetansky, M.D.)

There are many methods used in cleft palate repair. With some, the cleft is closed in one operation, and, with others, two procedures are needed. Like lip repair, the choice of procedure depends upon the surgeon and what he feels will be most successful in creating a competent velopharyngeal valve with minimal maxillary and dental deformities (43).

As with lip repair, there are differences of opinion as to when palate repair ought to take place. Most surgeons repair palates when the child is somewhere between twelve and twenty-four months of age. Those who advocate early repair feel that correct speech is more easily attained if the palate is repaired before a child begins talking. When surgery is delayed, the child learns to speak with a defective speech mechanism and compensates in such a way that correct speech after surgery will be difficult. It is felt, also, that early surgery reduces the amount of upper respiratory infections caused by the open palate (14, 36).

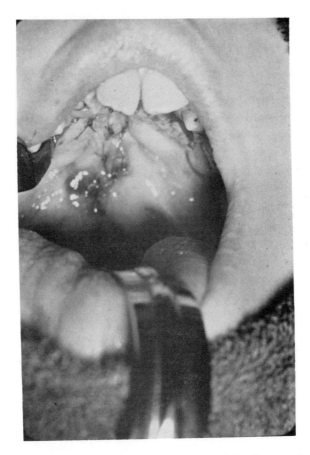

Figure 5. Repaired cleft palate. (Courtesy of D. Kapetansky, M.D.)

Approximately 60 percent of those who have a cleft palate acquire adequate speech after the initial palate repair. The remaining 40 percent, who do not acquire adequate speech, may do so following speech therapy, secondary surgery, or, as in most cases, a combination of both (5). The general aim of secondary surgery is to augment the soft palate in order to establish more adequate speech.

At present, the pharyngeal flap operation seems to be the most popular technique for the improvement of inadequate speech. This procedure involves the elevation of tissue from the wall of the pharynx leaving it attached either superiorly or inferiorly, swinging it across, and suturing it to the soft palate.

A recent modification of this principle has been reported by Kapetansky (17). His procedure involves the creation of two sections of tissue, one from each side of the pharynx, that are then brought together at the soft palate to create a single flap. This modification is known as the transverse pharyngeal flap procedure.

In summarizing, reconstructive surgery for the child with a cleft lip and palate begins with initial lip repair during the first six months of life. Secondary lip surgery takes place anytime thereafter through the teen years. The purpose of this secondary surgery is usually to improve the appearance of the lip and nose. The main purpose of palate surgery is to close the cleft in order to establish more efficient eating and speech. This repair is normally done between one and two years of age. Secondary surgery of the palate is sometimes necessary in order to improve closure and, therefore, to improve speech.

Chapter 5

DENTAL MANAGEMENT AND ITS

RELATIONSHIP TO SPEECH

THE DENTAL TEAM HAS AN IMPORTANT ROLE IN THE HABILITATION PROGRAM OF THE CHILD WITH A CLEFT PALATE and/or lip. An adequate dental staff usually consists of a skilled dentist, a trained orthodontist, and a prosthodontist. It is generally agreed that a significantly higher frequency of dental abnormalities occurs in those who have a cleft than in the general population (16).

Because the child with a cleft often has missing or malformed teeth, the role of general dentistry is a very important part of his care. There is an increase in tooth decay among children with clefts because of poor brushing habits, little attention to diet, and the general neglect of baby teeth because it is assumed that they are of very little value.

Contrary to this assumption, the first teeth are as important to general health and development of the jaws and facial bones as are the second teeth. In order to encourage normal growth of the jaw, it is important to preserve every tooth possible and to have each one grow as straight as possible. It is even more important to retain teeth in the case of a child with a cleft than in children without clefts because prosthetic and orthodontic devices may have to be attached to the teeth. With this in mind, it is advised that preventive dental care be initiated as early as three years of age.

Although it is generally agreed that the child with a cleft has more cavities than other children, this apparently does not have to be the case. In a study of 258 children with cleft palates, dental examinations showed that they did not have a significantly greater number of cavities than any other children (18). These results underscore the importance for good and consistent general dental care for the child with a cleft palate.

The orthodontist is concerned with the correction of irregularities of the teeth and jaws. His goal is to establish an occlusion that is acceptable in appearance and function. Since crooked teeth and malocclusions frequently accompany clefts, the orthodontist has much to contribute in the habilitation of the child.

Often an expansion appliance is needed to widen the palatal arch. These expansion bands vary, but basically consist of a curved wire that is fitted around the lingual aspect of the teeth and attached to the back teeth. Some orthodontists wait until the second teeth are in, but many prefer initiating treatment of this type at three or four years of age. Their opinion is that by establishing an acceptable occlusion of the baby teeth, the permanent teeth will be able to erupt in a more favorable position. Also, oral hygiene and periodontal conditions will be improved and the tongue may assume a more normal position allowing for more normal growth and development (25).

After a period of treatment, a retaining appliance is often inserted to maintain the correction. These appliances are usually thin shells of acrylic plastic molded to fit the palatal vault. If the patient lacks some teeth, they can be added to the retainer to improve appearance and speech (40).

Recently, orthodontic work has been initiated even before plastic surgery by fitting a simple orthodontic appliance in newborns. The purpose of this appliance is to control the alignment of the upper jaw segments. It is felt that there are real advantages to this early procedure. The appliance closes the hard palate so that normal feeding can be established shortly after birth. This should encourage the use of the tongue tip and reduce the tendency for the child to rely on the back of the tongue for later speech production. Other advantages are that it probably facilitates repair of the lip and promotes growth of the maxillary segments (24).

The role of the prosthodontist is to augment existing structures with bridges, dentures, and obturators (40). A patient may require a denture because of a residual palatal fistula or because of the absence of individual teeth either from the cleft or from the effect of dental decay. Where there is a fistula, the dental plate may be necessary to cover the aperture and prevent the leakage of air flow from the mouth into the nasal cavity. Even a small opening of this type may hinder the normal development of speech.

An obturator is a type of dental plate worn by the patient to form a roof to the mouth and cover the cleft. It can also be designed as a speech aid. It is sometimes used before surgery, sometimes in place of surgery, or sometimes with surgery to aid in reducing nasality in speech (24).

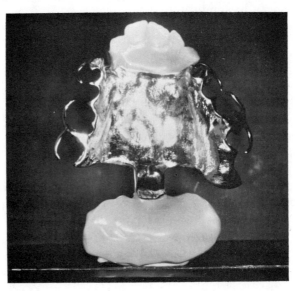

Figure 6. Prosthesis showing obturator and replacement dental units. (Courtesy of H. Metz, D.D.S.)

Some obturators have three parts: an anterior part that fits into the palatal vault, a middle part that connects the front and back parts, and a posterior part (bulb) that fills in the pharyngeal space behind the soft palate and closes the opening between the nasal and oral cavities. The muscles of the throat tighten around the margins of the bulb to seal off the nasal cavity. When they relax there is an opening large enough for nasal breathing and the production of nasal consonants. The appliance may, therefore, serve several purposes.

It can (a) improve the profile by supporting the upper lip, (b) supply missing teeth, (c) serve as a retainer to maintain orthodontic correction, (d) close openings in the hard palate, (e) improve occlusion, and (f) close the opening between the oral and nasal cavity (40).

Caruso (2) has indicated that when surgery is feasible, it is considered more economical than long-term use of an appliance, but, when there is insufficient tissue or when the patient is a poor surgical risk, an appliance may be the primary treatment choice.

The question occurs as to how much dental management affects the speech of a child with a cleft lip or palate. There are varying opinions as to the role of dental irregularities as a cause of speech defects in individuals without cleft palate. In a study that compared the articulation of several sounds between children whose incisor teeth were present and those whose incisors were missing, results showed that, for a few children, the condition of the teeth was a crucial factor in the development of correct articulation (30). However, the results also showed that defective incisors usually do not interfere with correct articulation. This is basically true for children with clefts too, except here the speech mechanism is already somewhat handicapped if there is insufficient velopharyngeal closure and is less able to compensate for dental deformities; therefore, most of these irregularities assume a greater significance (9).

During speech, the teeth provide a cutting edge for the impedance of the breath stream for various consonant sounds. If spaces exist that are so wide that the effects of the cutting edges are lost, then sounds such as the s, z, th, f, and v may be produced in a distorted manner.

Open bite is another fairly common dental deviation that in all probability may cause defectiveness of fricative sounds. Any irregularities in the teeth or arch that interfere with proper tongue placement can be a detriment to correct speech.

In conclusion, then, it would be justified to state that velopharyngeal closure is most important for good speech production, but that the teeth and dental arches are also important for correct articulation. The dental team, therefore, is a very important and necessary facet in the management of the child with a cleft lip and/or palate. The general dentist is important in preventing tooth decay of the child with a cleft. The orthodontist is necessary to correct improper occlusions, to provide an expansion appliance to widen the palatal arch, or to fit an orthodontic appliance in a newborn. The role of the prosthodontist is to augment the existing structures with bridges, dentures, and obturators. The obturator, often referred to as a speech aid, is sometimes used to cover the cleft, but may also extend into the velopharyngeal port in order to facilitate separation of the nasal and oral cavities for speech purposes.

Chapter 6

EMOTIONAL ADJUSTMENT OF THE

CHILD WITH A CLEFT LIP OR PALATE

OF PROBABLE CONCERN TO EVERY PARENT WHOSE BABY IS BORN WITH A CLEFT OF ANY TYPE IS HOW THIS IRREGULARITY will affect the child's later emotional adjustment. At present there are contrasting views regarding this aspect.

Many experienced clinicians agree that psychological problems do exist for these individuals. One speech clinician, known for her extensive work with cleft palate individuals, states:

It must be remembered that to the child with a cleft palate his speech is the same as that of the people around him, and he may reach the age of six, seven or even eight years before he is consciously able to recognize any difference, and then only through training. . . However, the child discovers that he differs from others in that he cannot make his speech intelligible to anyone, with the possible exception of his mother and his own family. It is here that he is faced with a problem which he is unable to solve without help. In the majority of these cases the results appear to be bewilderment and eventual acceptance of the fact that there is a difference between himself and others. There may be withdrawal from social contacts and a tendency to avoid speech, even refusal to speak at all, while in others a more aggressive attitude may develop. . . . Unless something is done to help the child to remedy the defect, matters will become worse as he grows older and develops an increasing sensitiveness to his abnormality. In many cases where operative procedures have been delayed normal self-confidence has been replaced by feelings of inferiority associated with a subconscious fear of speech, this condition being intensified by the fact that the patient has not the knowledge nor ability to do anything to remedy matters unaided (24, p. 221).

In agreement are other clinicians who state that speech difficulties and facial scars may cause some psychological and social maladjustments.

Ruess (27), a clinical psychologist, states that of all the dimensions of personality necessary for satisfactory and successful social interaction, facial configuration and oral communication are probably two of the most important. "Abnormality" of either may lead to social and personal maladjustment. He states, further, that for the cleft palate individual there are two possible dimensions most likely to affect his social interaction and, in effect, impose a handicap: inadequate speech and facial disfigurement.

Cleft palate children seem to have greater difficulty in the use of language and have less well-developed body-image concepts than would be expected among the general population with similar characteristics of age, sex, and intelligence. Numerous children without cleft palates, however, are also known to have deficiencies in one or two areas of language functioning and to have deficient body-image concepts.

Fischoff (10), in his experience with children with congenital handicaps, has found that the physiological stress these children are subjected to early in life can cause anxiety, a longer dependency period, and a defective body-image. He has observed that children with clefts often use defense mechanisms of denial, isolation, and reaction formation in dealing with their cleft.

Children with clefts have also been described as being shy, nervous, less aggressive, less confident, and less independent than their noncleft peers (21, 32).

In contrast to the assumptions of some clinicians, several studies of various psychosocial dimensions suggest little if any difference between children with clefts and their noncleft peers.

One such study (39) was conducted wherein boys with cleft lip and palate were given a personal adjustment inventory that consisted of reports of wishes, self-evaluations, likes, dislikes, and fantasies. Their scores were compared to those of boys without clefts. The results suggest that no significant differences existed between the two groups of boys.

In a similar study (28), children with clefts were evaluated for social adjustment with a series of personality tests. Again, the results did not lend support to the assumption that the social adjustment of cleft palate children is markedly inferior to that of other children.

In a study (8) of the high school dropout rate for cleft palate patients, no relationship could be established between the type of cleft or presence of a speech and hearing impairment and the factor of nongraduation from high school. The cleft palate subjects who dropped out of high school were not necessarily those with more involved clefts, more severe speech problems, or greater hearing loss. In families where the siblings graduated from high school, an overwhelming number of cleft palate subjects also graduated.

In a more recent study, selected personality traits of children with clefts were compared to their siblings. Results indicated no significant difference between the two groups in personality and adjustment (42).

Adults with repaired clefts have been found to be generally satisfied with their bodies and themselves when compared to noncleft adults, although less satisfied with their mouth, teeth, and speech than with other characteristics. Many of the adults reported that their social life, personality, and career were not affected by the cleft (4, 26).

Parent reactions such as shock, rejection, guilt, and overprotection can influence the parent-child relationship and adjustment of the child. Although these reactions to the birth of a child with a cleft are quite normal, they may have a negative effect on the child's psychosocial development if they are not resolved.

Early family counseling is a vital part of the habilitation program of the child with a cleft. Early counseling can help the parents understand the nature of their child's handicap, their own feelings, and can help the child to develop confidence and self-acceptance.

In summarizing, research shows two distinct opinions regarding the social and emotional adjustment of those with clefts. Clinicians state from experience that these children are often withdrawn and shy due to their speech difficulties and facial disfigurements. Results of studies, on the other hand, have found no significant differences in the emotional and social adjustment between those with clefts and those without clefts. It seems safe to assume that a child with a cleft who has received good medical care and has established fairly normal speech will not experience any serious personality problems if the psychosocial aspects of the cleft are appropriately handled.

Chapter 7

AUDITORY MANAGEMENT FOR THE

CHILD WITH A CLEFT PALATE

F OR THE PAST SEVERAL YEARS THERE HAS BEEN A GROWING INTEREST IN THE RELATIONSHIP BETWEEN HEARING loss and the cleft palate and/or lip. A number of studies (13, 15, 19, 23, 29) have been carried out to determine just how many children with clefts also suffer from hearing losses. Research findings have indicated that from 19 percent to 62 percent of children with clefts also have hearing losses.

This disagreement in exact percentages may be because there has been no set standard for defining a hearing loss. Each examiner or researcher has set his own decibel and frequency standard for what he feels constitutes a hearing loss (33).

For the purposes of this discussion it would be safe to state that approximately 50 percent of all children with cleft palate and lip suffer from some hearing loss. This is considerably higher than the 3 to 4 percent hearing loss in normal schoolchildren (40).

There has been widespread agreement that these losses are generally mild to moderate in degree; are bilateral, that is, occurring in both ears; and are usually of the conductive type (13, 23, 29, 44). The word *conductive* is used to denote a problem in the middle portion of the ear. This is opposed to other types of hearing loss, such as when the nerves are damaged.

There have been efforts to establish whether hearing loss is more prevalent in certain types of clefts; whether the type of management, be it surgical or prosthetic, is significant; and whether age at the time of palate repair is in any way related to the hearing loss. At this time there has been no real indication that any of these factors cause a greater incidence of hearing loss.

An extensive study has been reported by Skolnik (29). His research was carried out over eight years with 401 individuals with cleft lip and palate. He found that 30 percent of the 401 had some hearing loss. He broke this down into age groups and found that 6 percent of those children under one year of age had a loss; 27 percent of the one-to-four-year-old group had a hearing loss; and 68 percent of the five-to-thirteen-year-old group had hearing loss. He attributed this large increase from preschool to school age children to contagious diseases as well as to the increased incidence of upper respiratory infections a child encounters once he starts school.

In this particular study, no relationship could be found between type of cleft and hearing loss, although it has been found, in other studies, that more hearing losses occur with clefts of the palate only (22, 33, 35). Skolnik also found that there was no sex prevalence in the frequency of ear pathology in cleft palate patients; hearing loss was mild in more than one-half the cases, moderate in about one-quarter, and severe in about 4 percent; and early closure did not reduce the incidence of ear pathology.

The occurrence of hearing loss in the cleft palate population is due to the increased number of middle-ear disorders that occur within this group. Such disorders occur because the eustachian tube does not normally open and close in order to keep the middle ear dry. The fluid may be infectious or noninfectious, but its presence nevertheless results in hearing loss. It is felt that the best way to avoid hearing loss with a cleft palate child is to have good medical attention with the parent reporting any minor ear problems to the doctor to avoid further complications. It can be speculated that if this would be done a great many hearing losses could be avoided (15).

The child's ability to recognize and interpret sound, which eventually leads to speech, develops primarily during the first year of life. Since speech development is based upon adequate reception of speech sounds, adequate hearing, especially up to the age of two years, becomes extremely important. Diagnosis of a hearing problem as early as possible is essential in all children; it is even more essential in a child with a cleft palate, who has a potential speech problem due to the cleft.

Failure to recognize and promptly treat a hearing problem will greatly handicap the child's entire speech habilitation program (41). A severe hearing defect will prevent the imitation of speech and cause severe delay and a limitation in the use of speech. Where the hearing loss is partial, the child will not hear the sounds of speech normally. Consonant sounds may be distorted, and he will reproduce them as he hears them (24). There may be reduced ability in oral communication, vocabulary, and grammar as well.

There are several things that the parent can watch for at home that might give a clue as to just how well the young child is hearing.

1. Does the infant's hearing seem normal?

2. Does he appear to respond to sound, especially to the mother's voice, by turning or smiling, or reaching toward her?

3. Does he make an effort to produce sound himself? Babbling in early months and disappearance of these sounds at approximately nine months, with no further speech development, would suggest a hearing impairment.

4. Does the child seem unaware of activities, especially those associated with sound, taking place around him?

5. Does the child have unexplained crying spells as if he were in pain or frequent pulling on the ear lobe indicating possible earaches? (41, p. 206).

In conclusion, approximately 50 percent of all children with cleft palate and lip suffer from hearing loss as compared to 3 to 4 percent hearing loss in normal schoolchildren. The hearing loss of this 50 percent is usually mild to moderate and is felt to be caused, in many instances, by respiratory infections. It is the opinion of many that prompt medical care can aid a great deal in reducing hearing losses among cleft palate children.

Chapter **8**

TECHNIQUES TO ASSIST IN SPEECH

AND LANGUAGE DEVELOPMENT

QUESTIONS REGARDING SPEECH AND LANGUAGE DEVELOPMENT ARE OFTEN OF MAJOR CONCERN TO PARENTS OF THE cleft palate baby. How will the cleft affect speech; when should speech therapy begin; and what can they do to help their child's speech to appropriately develop? In order to answer these questions, this chapter will present a summary of speech and language development; a description of speech and language problems related to the cleft palate and lip; and suggestions to stimulate the speech and language development of a child with an oral cleft.

Speech and Language Development

Although a child usually begins talking between one and two years of age, prespeech activities that are crucial in the process of speech and language development begin much sooner than that. They can be said to begin at birth with the first cry of the infant.

The acquisition of speech and language is a highly complex and impressive process involving several components and would take a rather lengthy textbook to describe in detail.

Two major components of the process of communication, however, consist of language and speech. The term *language* may be thought of as the understanding or comprehension of a message that is being communicated through listening or reading (receptive language) and the ability to express one's thoughts and ideas through talking and writing (expressive language). The term *speech* is defined as the ability to vocalize and pronounce (articulate) sounds and, to combine these sounds in such a way as to form words. Speech is actually the final phase of expressive language, and can be considered the mechanical portion of talking.

Language acquisition is dependent upon a person's ability to hear the speech of others, interpret what is being said, and to retrieve from memory the appropriate words to respond expressively to the message. Speech is dependent upon the ability to vocalize sound in the larynx and, then, to form that sound into individual vowels and consonants with the tongue, lips, and teeth. For example, if someone asked you what movie you would like to see, you would have to have the hearing acuity necessary to hear the question, and you would need to have the comprehension skills necessary to understand what the spoken words meant. Then, in order to respond, you would have to recall the words that properly answer the question and, finally, form those chosen words with the speech mechanism to express your answer.

Obviously, children are not born with the ability to understand or speak a language. Prespeech activities, those that prepare the child for later communication, do, however, begin in early infancy when the child cries and, a few months later, starts to coo and babble, thus producing various consonant and vowel sounds. Although not usually thought of in terms of speech, eating is also a valuable prespeech activity because the child uses the same musculature in sucking and chewing that will be used later in articulating words. During feeding, the baby is exercising and learning to coordinate lip and tongue movements that are very significant in producing the individual speech sounds.

By approximately six months of age, most children have reached what is referred to as the "babbling" stage. During this stage, babies vocalize and experiment with sound. This babbling consists of repetitions of sounds and syllables such as "buh-buh" and "guh-guh-guh." This particular phase of development is considered to be a very important part of speech and language development and should be encouraged by parents. Parents can stimulate babbling by talking to their baby and by giving the baby some opportunity to be alone and to babble uninterruptedly. Children who receive verbal stimulation from adults have been found to babble more than those who are brought up in an environment that lacks this type of stimulation. It has also been found that babies have a tendency to stop babbling when they hear another person's voice. For this reason, it is advised that the baby be given some time alone to enjoy and experiment with his sound-making.

Between nine and twelve months of age, a child begins to echo words that he hears such as "ma-ma" and "bye-bye." Usually, these words do not have any meaning to the child, but are an imitation of what he hears.

At some point between twelve and eighteen months (there is a great deal of variation between children), the child begins to say his first true words in a meaningful way. At this point he has become a communicating individual and is learning to express his needs and wants through language. It is important to note here that, although the child has started to say words, they are not necessarily articulated correctly; "cookie" may sound more like "kuh-kuh" and "water" may be pronounced "wawa" or "wuh."

Receptive language also begins to develop early in infancy and is usually more developed than expressive language when compared at the same age. For example, a child of approximately ten months may not be saying words, but will understand simple requests such as "Show me your nose" and "Where's your shoe?"

Receptive language begins to develop when the infant responds to voices by turning his head toward the source of the sound; at this point, he is developing what is known as auditory awareness. Soon, he begins to recognize his mother's voice from all others, and the discrimination of auditory signals is starting. Sometime during the last half of his first year, the baby begins to understand some words such as "no," "cookie," "bottle," and will begin to respond to his name.

When a child begins to speak, he uses single-word utterances such as "allgone," "there," and "ball," to get his message across. A single-word utterance can have several different meanings. "Doggy" can mean "I see a doggy," "Where is the doggy?," or any four-legged creature with fur.

At the next phase of development, the child begins to put two words together such as " Where daddy?," "More cookie," "Mommy shoe." At the same time, he is beginning to comprehend more and more around him and gradually begins to use longer sentences and more complex grammar.

The experiences a child has and the knowledge he has of the world around him are very important for the development of speech and language skills. Of equal importance is having someone to talk to and feeling the need to communicate.

Speech and Language Problems
Related to the Cleft Palate and Lip

Not all children with a cleft of the lip and/or palate have the same type of speech and language difficulties or the same degree of severity. A baby with a cleft lip only will probably not demonstrate a speech disorder related to this type of cleft.

Some children have very little difficulty with speech and language, while others are very difficult to understand. Fortunately, the prognosis for normal or near normal speech and language is usually very good if the child receives appropriate medical, dental, and speech therapy services early in life.

Two of the most distinctive characteristics of speech frequently associated with cleft palate are nasal emission of sounds and inappropriate articulation.

Nasal emission is present before the palate is repaired because the child is unable to close the opening between the oral and nasal cavities. This is normally accomplished by the soft palate moving up and back to meet the pharyngeal wall (wall of the throat). Since the child's palate has a cleft, he is not able to make a closure that divides the oral and nasal cavities; consequently, air is able to pass through to the nasal cavity instead of being directed through the oral cavity. This nasal emission often continues after surgery because the child has not learned to direct the airflow through the mouth.

Inappropriate articulation is also a major factor contributing to the unintelligible speech frequently heard in the child with a cleft. These errors can be the result of one or a combination of several causes.

During the first two years of life when the child is developing speech and language, the palate is often still unrepaired. In an attempt to close that opening, the child has a tendency to hold the tongue back in the mouth. As a result, several sounds that are normally produced by the tongue-tip are produced incorrectly at the back of the mouth.

Problems associated with the relationship between the upper and lower jaws and misaligned teeth that frequently accompany a cleft of the palate and lip, as well as inadequate lip movement, can also be contributing factors in articulation difficulties. If the jaws are not in proper alignment, it is sometimes difficult for the child to produce such sounds as s, z, sh, ch, and j. If it is difficult for the child to close his lips, the p, b, and m may be distorted.

Hearing loss is also a cause that needs to be considered with regard to the misarticulations that accompany a cleft. As stated in Chapter VII, it has been found that there is a greater than average incidence of hearing loss in the cleft-palate population. This is because children with clefts are more prone to ear infections than most children.

If the child has a hearing loss, even intermittently, during the years that speech and language are developing, he will not be hearing the sounds of speech correctly, and, therefore, will not be able to appropriately imitate them.

Several studies in recent years have investigated the receptive and expressive language skills of children with clefts. It has been found that the ability of these children to comprehend what is being communicated to them is well within normal range. When a problem in receptive language has been found, it has usually been attributed to an earlier hearing loss.

Research has indicated that the expressive skills of this population are slightly reduced when compared to children without clefts. There are several reasons that may account for this reduction in expressive language skills.

A hearing loss at an early age may affect the development of expressive language just as it may affect comprehension and articulation skills.

Another factor that may contribute to reduced expressive language skills is the reaction of the child or his parents to his unintelligible speech. Oftentimes, a child who is difficult to understand senses this inadequacy and will refrain from talking as much as possible or will revert to gestures. The parents of a child with a cleft, due to their inability to understand his speech, may anticipate the child's needs rather than requiring him to use language.

Language, like any other skill, only improves with use. Just as a golfer will not improve his score if he only golfs a few times a season, so the child will not improve his linguistic skills if he does not have the opportunity or feel the need to use language.

Suggestions to Stimulate Speech and Language Development

Ideally, the child with a cleft palate should come in contact with the speech and language pathologist as early in infancy as possible. The speech pathologist can be a valuable source of information for the parent regarding "typical" speech and langauge development and can periodically assess the language development of the child, initiate a home program to stimulate language skills, and determine when formal speech therapy should begin. Since prespeech skills begin to develop in early infancy, speech and language stimulation from the parent should also begin early in the child's life.

As stated earlier, a child usually reaches the "babbling" stage at about six months of age. Since this is such an important stage in language development, it is important that the parent encourage the child to babble by talking to him and by imitating the sounds that the baby makes. By imitating the child's vocalizations, the parent can frequently get the baby to imitate in return.

Before a child can learn to talk, he must associate objects and actions with a spoken word and understand that words have meaning. In order for this comprehension of language to develop, the young child needs to hear a word over and over many times. From the time he is approximately six or seven months of age, the parent should make it a point to name objects and actions that the child is involved with. For instance, when being given his ball, the child should hear the word "ball" so that he will begin to associate the word with the round object that he likes to play with on the floor.

As the child gets older, the parent can help in vocabulary development by giving him a variety of experiences that expose him to the world around him. These experiences do not require that the parent plan specific activities to develop their child's language, but rather can be part of the typical family routine. Everyday family activities are probably the greatest source of learning for the child if one takes advantage of them.

For example, a trip to the grocery store can give the child an opportunity to hear the names of various products, and also give him an opportunity to practice naming these items. If the child is older, the parent can talk to him about the differences between items, e.g. fruits vs. vegetables, food items vs. paper products, etc., and point out the sizes and shapes of the various items being purchased. The following is an example of the variety of vocabulary and concepts that the child can be exposed to through this experience: "This is a *big* can, and this is a *little* can." "The soup is in a *red* can, can you find it?" "The crackers are in a *box*; is this juice in a *box*?" "Do you remember what we call the thing that the juice comes in?" "The oranges are *round*; can you find something else that's *round*?"

As one can foresee, not only does this type of experience help the child to learn the names of objects, but can also provide a source for introducing him to the concepts of shape, color, number, and classification.

An example of another experience might be baking cookies. By allowing the child to participate and talking to him about what is being done, he will again be introduced to new vocabulary and concepts. He can be exposed to terms such as stir, mix, measure, pour, bake, flour, sugar, salt, etc. This can be an ideal time to talk about the differences in the way foods taste, using sugar and salt as an example, or to call his attention to the fact that the "flour" you are using for the cooking is different from the "flowers" that grow outside even though they sound the same.

After the cookies are baked, a discussion of what was done provides a good opportunity for the child to use language. The following is an example of the types of questions that may be used to elicit conversation from the child: "What did we do *first*?" "Do you remember what *ingredients* we needed?" "Remember we had to mix the flour and sugar;

were the cookies done then?" "What did we have to do *next*?" "*Why* did we put them in the oven?"

Words become a part of a child's vocabulary much sooner if he has actually experienced the activity and touched and used the objects involved. As one can realize from the two situations cited, typical everyday activities can provide an excellent source for language stimulation if the advantage is taken.

Simple games can also be created that help the child to develop language concepts. For instance, a game can be made from having the child follow directions, such as "Put the ball *between* the blocks." Guessing games can be played that teach color, shape, and functions of objects, such as, "I spy something *green*;" or, "I see something *round that we use to tell time with*."

It is important to provide children with an opportunity to use language. On the other hand, it is very easy in our busy hectic lives to talk to children rather than to communicate with them.

Providing an opportunity to use language can be created in just the way a question is asked. For example, "Do you want to wear your red shirt or your green shirt?" requires a response from the child of "my red one" or "red", as opposed to the question "Do you want to wear your red shirt," which requires only a yes or no response. "Do you want cereal or eggs?" requires, again, that the child say a word other than yes or no, or to nod his head. By wording questions in such a way, the child is provided with an opportunity to use the language he knows, and he will begin to realize what a valuable skill it is.

It is well-known that children do not generally pronounce words perfectly when they first begin to speak. The child with a cleft palate and lip usually has even more difficulty than most children because of his inappropriate use of the tongue and lips in articulation. When the child begins to talk, it is important that the parent not correct him or ask him to repeat words over and over again. The child, at this point, is speaking in the best way he knows and continual criticism could very well cause him to avoid talking whenever possible.

Instead, parents can stimulate improved sound production by devising games whereby their child can imitate the sounds parents make. The parent might play a sound version of Simon Says, such as "Simon says to do this, t-t-t"; or "Simon says to do this, mmmmm." The child should be shown where to put his tongue for the t sound and to put his lips together for the m.

Children are great imitators and love to mimic. Any type of activity that will teach them to move their lips and tongue will improve the oral-motor movements necessary for good articulation.

Good listening skills are also an important part of speech and language development. A youngster must first become aware of sound, then learn to discriminate between various sounds, and finally be able to comprehend what has been spoken. Since children born with a cleft palate have been found to have a higher incidence of hearing loss than the general population, activities to enhance listening skills are a very valuable part of their early experiences.

These skills can be strengthened in a variety of ways through books, records, nursery rhymes, and songs, as well as something as simple as calling the child's attention to the sounds around him.

A young child may find it difficult to follow a story that is read to him. However, even very young children enjoy looking through picture books while mom or dad name the pictures or tell a simplified version of the story.

In order for a child to be able to learn to produce the various sounds used in speech and to put sounds together to form words, he has to learn to discriminate between the individual sounds. Sometime during his development he will have to acquire the skill to recognize the difference between s and t, sh and ch, etc., and recognize that there is a difference between the words "bat" and "cat," "house" and "horse," etc.

This ability to discriminate between sounds, like all speech and language skills, has its beginning at an early age when the infant first differentiates the sound of his mother's voice from other voices. Slowly, this ability to discriminate becomes more and more sophisticated to the point that the child can recognize very slight differences between individual sounds.

Activities can be created that increase the child's awareness of different sounds in the environment, such as a dog barking, a bird chirping or the sound of a fire engine siren, bulldozer, or a doorbell. Games that require the child to guess the source of a sound can be played. While the child's eyes are closed, the parent can do such things as snap his fingers, crumple paper, tap a table, or ring a bell.

As the child becomes more adept at hearing differences between sounds, games can be played with the individual speech sounds. The parent can make two sounds such as m-m or m-b and the child can guess whether they were the same or different.

Suggestions for listening activities are virtually endless. The important thing to remember is that any activity or experience that requires the child to listen will be valuable in developing auditory skills.

Hopefully, the information in this chapter has given a better understanding of how speech and language develop and how your child can be helped to develop these skills.

The suggestions included here are meant to be just a beginning; it is anticipated that parents will be able to create numerous situations that will enhance the communication skills of their child.

In closing, it needs to be stressed that at no time should a parent drill on speech with their child. Make speech and language fun for the child and he will respond beautifully. If the activity is enjoyable for the parent, the parent can be sure that the child is also having a good time.

BIBLIOGRAPHY

1. Bzoch, Kenneth R.: Articulation proficiency and error patterns of preschool cleft palate and normal children. *Cleft Palate J,* 2:340-349, 1965.
2. Caruso, Anthony C.: Prosthodontics. In Stark, Richard B. (Ed.): *Cleft Palate: A Multidiscipline Approach.* New York, Harper & Row, 1968.
3. Chesky, R.: The role of the pediatrician in cleft palate management. In Falk, M. (Ed.): *A Cleft Palate Team Addresses the Speech Clinician.* Springfield, Charles C Thomas Publisher, 1971.

4. Clifford, E., Crocker, E., and Pope, G.: Psychological findings in the adulthood of 98 cleft lip and cleft palate children. *Plastic and Reconstructive Surgery, 50*:234-237, 1972.

5. Converse, John Marquis: The techniques of cleft palate surgery. In ASHA Reports, No. 1: *Proceedings of the Conference: Communicative Problems in Cleft Palate,* 1965.

6. Counihan, Donald T.: Articulation skills of adolescents and adults with cleft palates. *J Speech Hearing Dis, 25*:181-187, 1960.

7. Dehaan, Clayton R.: Initial repair of cleft lip. In Stark, Richard B. (Ed.): *Cleft Palate: A Multidiscipline Approach.* New York, Harper & Row, 1968.

8. Demb, Norman, and Ruess, Aubrey, L.: High school dropout for cleft palate patients. *Cleft Palate J, 4*:327-33, 1967.

9. Drillien, Cecil M., Ingram, T.T.S., and Wilkinson, Elsie M.: *The Causes and Natural History of Cleft Lip and Palate.* Baltimore, Williams & Wilkins, 1966.

10. Fischoff, J.: Psychiatric considerations of the cleft palate child. In Falk, M. (Ed.): *A Cleft Palate Team Addresses the Speech Clinician.* Springfield, Charles C Thomas Publisher, 1971.

11. Fogh-Anderson, P.: Epidemiology and etiology of clefts. In Bergsma, D. (Ed.): *Birth Defects.* Baltimore, Williams and Wilkins, 1971.

12. Fogh-Anderson, P.: Incidence and aetiology. In Edwards, M. and Watson, A.C.H. (Eds.): *Advances in the Management of Cleft Palate.* New York, Churchill Livingstone, 1980.

13. Halfond, Murray M., and Ballenger, John J.: An audiologic and otorhinologic study of cleft lip and cleft palate cases: I audiologic evaluation. *Arch Otolaryng (Chicago) 64*:58-62, 1956.

14. Holdsworth, W.G.: *Cleft Lip and Palate,* 2nd ed. London, Grune, 1957.

15. Holmes, Edgar M., and Reed, George F.: Hearing and deafness in cleft palate patients. *Arch Otolaryng* (Chicago), *62*:620-24, 1955.

16. Jordan, Ronald E., Krause, Bertram S., and Neptune, C. Marshall: Dental abnormalities associated with cleft lip and/or palate. *Cleft Palate J, 3*:22-55, 1966.

17. Kapetansky, D.I.: Bilateral transverse pharyngeal flaps for repair of cleft palate. *Journal of Plastic and Reconstructive Surgery, 52*:52-54, 1973.

18. Lauterstein, Aubrey M., and Mendelsohn, Mark: An analysis of the caries experience of 258 cleft palate children. *Cleft Palate J, 1*:314-19, 1964.

19. MacCollum, Donald W., and Richardson, Sylvia Onesti: Management of the patient with cleft lip and cleft palate. *Pediatrics, 20*:573-584, 1957.

20. McWilliams, Betty Jane: Articulation problems of a group of cleft palate adults. *J Speech Hearing Res, 1*:68-74, 1958.

21. McWilliams, B.J., and Musgrave, R.H.: Psychological implications of articulation disorders of cleft palate children. *Cleft Palate Journal, 9*:294-303, 1972.

22. Masters, F.W., Bingham, H.G., and Robinson, D.W.: The prevention and treatment of hearing loss in the cleft palate child. *Plast Reconstr Surg, 25*:503-09, 1960.

23. Miller, Maurice H.: Hearing losses in cleft palate cases. *Laryngoscope, 66*:1492-96, 1956.

24. Morley, Muriel E.: *Cleft Palate and Speech,* 7th ed. London, Churchill Livingstone, 1970.

25. Olin, William H.: *Cleft Lip and Palate Rehabilitation.* Springfield, Charles C Thomas Publisher, 1960.

26. Pickerell, K., *et al.*: Study of 100 cleft lip-palate patients operated upon 22 to 27 years ago by one surgeon. *Plastic and Reconstructive Surgery. 49*:149-155, 1972.

27. Ruess, A.L.: The clinical psychologist in habilitation of the cleft palate patient. *J Speech Hearing Dis, 23*:561-76, 1958.

28. Sidney, Ruth Ann, and Matthews, Jack: An evaluation of the social adjustment of a group of cleft palate children. *Cleft Palate Bull, 6*:10, 1956.

29. Skolnik, Emanuel M.: Otologic evaluation in cleft palate patients. *Laryngoscope, 68*:1908-49, 1958.

30. Snow, Katherine: Articulation proficiency in relation to certain dental abnormalities. *J Speech Hearing Dis, 26*:209-12, 1961.

31. Spriestersbach, D.C.: The effects of orofacial anomalies on the speech process. *Proceedings of the Conference: Communicative Problems in Cleft Palate.* ASHA Reports, No. 1, pp. 111-28, 1965.

32. Spriestersbach, D.C.: *Psychosocial Aspects of the Cleft Palate Problem.* Iowa City, University of Iowa, 1973.

33. Spriestersbach, D.C. *et al.*: Hearing loss in children with cleft palates. *Plas Reconstr Surg, 30*:336-47, 1962.

34. Spriestersbach, D.C., Darley, Fredric L., and Rouse, Verna: Articulation of a group of children with cleft lips and palates. *J Speech Hearing Dis, 21*:436-45, 1956.

35. Spriestersbach, D.C., Moll, Kenneth L., and Morris, Hughlett L.: Heterogeneity of the 'cleft palate population' and research design. *Cleft Palate J, 1*:210-16, 1964.

36. Stark, Richard B.: Initial repair of cleft palate. In Stark, Richard B. (Ed.): *Cleft Palate: A Multidiscipline Approach.* New York, Harper & Row, 1968.

37. Stark, Richard B.: Secondary repair of cleft lip. In Stark, Richard B. (Ed.): *Cleft Palate: A Multidiscipline Approach.* New York, Harper & Row, 1968.

38. Steigler, Eleanor J., and Berry, Mildred F.: A new look at the etiology of cleft palate. *Plast Reconstr Surg, 21*:52-73, 1958.

39. Watson, Charles G.: Personality adjustment in boys with cleft lips and palates. *Cleft Palate J, 1*:130-38, 1964.

40. Westlake, Harold, and Rutherford, David: *Cleft Palate.* Englewood Cliffs, Prentice-Hall, 1966.

41. Whitefield, Stanley: Hearing evaluation. In Stark, Richard B. (Ed.): *Cleft Palate: A Multidiscipline Approach.* New York, Harper & Row, 1968.

42. Wirls, C.J., and Plotkin, R.R.: A comparison of children with cleft palate and their siblings on projective test personality factors. *Cleft Palate Journal, 8*:399-407, 1971.

43. Yules, R.B.: *Atlas for Surgical Repair of Cleft Lip, Cleft Palate and Noncleft Velopharyngeal Incompetence.* Springfield, Charles C Thomas Publisher, 1971.

44. Zimmerman, Jane Dorsey, and Canfield, William H.: Language and speech development. In Stark, Richard B. (Ed.): *Cleft Palate: A Multidiscipline Approach.* New York, Harper & Row, 1968.